Workbook to Accompany
Human Diseases
SECOND EDITION

Workbook to Accompany
Human Diseases
SECOND EDITION

MARIANNE NEIGHBORS, EdD, RN
Professor
Eleanor Mann School of Nursing
University of Arkansas
Fayetteville, Arkansas

RUTH TANNEHILL-JONES, MS, RN
Vice President, Patient Care Services
Chief Nurse Executive
St Mary's – Mercy Health System NW Arkansas

Written by
SANDRA LEHRKE, MS, RN
Medical Assistant Program Director
Anoka Technical College
Anoka, Minnesota

THOMSON

DELMAR LEARNING Australia Canada Mexico Singapore Spain United Kingdom United States

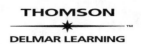

THOMSON

DELMAR LEARNING

Workbook to Accompany Human Diseases, Second Edition
Marianne Neighbors and Ruth Tannehill-Jones

Vice President, Health Care Business Unit:
William Brottmiller

Acquisitions Editor:
Marah Bellegarde

Editorial Assistant:
Jadin Babin-Kavanaugh

Developmental Editor:
Debra Flis

Marketing Director:
Jennifer McAvey

Health Care Channel Manager – Education:
Tamara Caruso

Marketing Coordinator:
Michele Gleason

Production Manager:
Barbara A. Bullock

Art & Design Coordinator:
Alexandros Vasilakos

Production Coordinator:
Thomas Heffernan

Project Editor:
Ruth Fisher

Library of Congress Cataloging-in-Publication Data:
ISBN 13: 978-1-4018-7089-8
ISBN 10: 1-4018-7089-9
CIP: 2005049726

NOTICE TO THE READER

Contents

Introduction   ix

UNIT I
Concepts of Human Diseases

CHAPTER 1
Introduction to Human Diseases   1

CHAPTER 2
Mechanisms of Disease   4

CHAPTER 3
Neoplasms   9

CHAPTER 4
Inflammation and Infection   16

UNIT II
Common Diseases and Disorders of Body Systems

CHAPTER 5
Immune System Diseases and Disorders   25

CHAPTER 6
Musculoskeletal System
Diseases and Disorders   37

CHAPTER 7
Blood and Blood-Forming Organs
Diseases and Disorders   **58**

CHAPTER 8
Cardiovascular System Diseases and Disorders   **71**

CHAPTER 9
Respiratory System Diseases and Disorders   **78**

CHAPTER 10
Lymphatic System Diseases and Disorders   **86**

CHAPTER 11
Digestive System Diseases and Disorders   **90**

CHAPTER 12
Liver, Gallbladder, and Pancreas
Diseases and Disorders   **97**

CHAPTER 13
Urinary System Diseases and Disorders   **102**

CHAPTER 14
Endocrine System Diseases and Disorders   **108**

CHAPTER 15
Nervous System Diseases and Disorders   **116**

CHAPTER 16
Eye and Ear Diseases and Disorders   **124**

CHAPTER 17
Reproductive System Diseases and Disorders   **131**

CHAPTER 18
Integumentary System Diseases
and Disorders   **139**

UNIT III
Genetic/Developmental, Childhood, and Mental Health Diseases and Disorders

CHAPTER 19
Genetic and Developmental
Diseases and Disorders   **148**

CHAPTER 20
Childhood Diseases and Disorders   **154**

CHAPTER 21
Mental Health Diseases and Disorders   **159**

Human Diseases, Second Edition, helps you learn basic disease information. Organized by body systems, this essential pathophysiology text is written specifically for allied health learners and as a reference for allied health professionals. This book is also ideal as a resource on basic diseases by anyone within the medical arena or lay community. It is designed to make difficult pathophysiology concepts easier to understand by using consistent organization, and it includes pronunciations, boxed features, and full-color illustrations and photos. Chapters progress through a basic review of anatomy and physiology before introducing the most common diseases. Common diseases and disorders are presented consistently through etiology, symptoms, and treatment headings.

TO THE LEARNER

Each chapter in the workbook corresponds to the same chapter in the book. A variety of exercises is included to help reinforce the material you learned in the book. Types of exercises include completion, short answer, case studies, defining terms, defining abbreviations, matching, and condition tables.

HUMAN DISEASES, SECOND EDITION, STUDYWARE™

Gain additional practice with the Study-Ware™ CD-ROM that offers an exciting way to enhance your learning of human diseases. The quizzes and activities are an interactive and engaging way to reinforce the content in the book. Review the *How to Use Human Diseases, Second Edition, StudyWare™* in your book for a detailed description of this component.

Introduction to Human Diseases

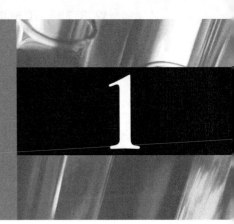

1

COMPLETION

Using the words in the list, complete the following statements:

disease	homeostasis	disorder	syndrome
pathology	pathologist	pathogens	pathogenesis
acute	chronic	etiology	idiopathic
iatrogenic	nosocomial	predisposing factors	diagnosis
symptoms	auscultation	palpation	percussion
prognosis	remission	exacerbations	complication
signs	mortality	fatal	holistic medicine
preventive	palliative	lethal	

1. _____ care is aimed at preventing pain and discomfort but does not seek to cure the disease.

2. The state of sameness or normalcy is known as _____.

3. _____ is the study of disease.

4. A time when symptoms are diminished or temporarily resolved is called _____.

5. A condition that is short term with a sudden onset is called _____.

6. A change in structure or function within the body that is considered abnormal is known as _____.

7. A deadly disease is called _____ or _____.

8. A problem arising from a prescribed treatment is called _____.

9. Risk factors are also called _____ _____.

10. The cause of disease is _____.

11. _____ is the predicted or expected outcome.

12. _____, _____, and _____
are used during a physical examination.

13. _____ are the problems a patient reports to the physician.

14. Flare-ups or return of symptoms are _____.

15. When the physician identifies or names a disease, he or she is making a
_____.

16. The _____ are what the physician sees or measures during an
examination.

17. Diabetes is a _____ disease because it lasts for a long or extended
period of time.

18. A disease acquired from the hospital environment is called _____.

19. The concept where the whole person, rather than just the physical being, is considered is
known as _____ medicine.

20. A group of symptoms that may be caused by several interrelated problems is known as a
_____.

SHORT ANSWER

Answer the following questions:

1. Define *predisposing factors*.

_____

_____

_____

2. List the predisposing factors.

a. _____

b. _____

c. _____

d. _____

e. _____

3. List possible treatment interventions.

   a. _____

   b. _____

   c. _____

   d. _____

4. Give four examples of preventive treatments.

   a. _____

   b. _____

   c. _____

   d. _____

CASE STUDY

Emily is a 25-year-old Asian female. Emily is complaining of frequent headaches over the past 3 weeks. Emily is taking birth control pills and smokes one package of cigarettes a day. She complains of severe head pain, light sensitivity, nausea, and vomiting. She has had no relief from over-the-counter medications such as Tylenol or ibuprofen.

Using the information from the case study, list a possible diagnosis, risk factors, symptoms, and the etiology.

_____

_____

_____

_____

_____

_____

2 Mechanisms of Disease

DEFINING TERMS

Define the following terms:

1. congenital _____

2. infection _____

3. hyperplasia _____

4. neoplasm _____

5. oncology _____

6. malignant _____

7. benign _____

8. cancer _____

9. metastatic _____

10. parenteral _____

11. degeneration _____

_____

12. hypertrophy _____

_____

13. atrophy _____

_____

14. ischemia _____

_____

15. gangrene _____

_____

16. infarct _____

_____

17. hypoxia _____

_____

18. antibodies _____

_____

19. total parenteral nutrition _____

_____

20. cachexia _____

_____

SHORT ANSWER

Describe the following causes of disease and give an example of each:

1. heredity

_____

_____

_____

2. trauma

_____

_____

_____

3. inflammation/infection

_____

_____

_____

4. hyperplasias/neoplasms

_____

_____

_____

5. nutritional imbalance

_____

_____

_____

6. malnutrition

_____

_____

_____

7. impaired immunity

_____

_____

_____

SHORT ANSWER

Answer the following questions:

1. What are the common ways the immune system may malfunction?

_____

_____

_____

2. List two ways the immune system protects the body.

_____

_____

_____

3. What factors affect the aging process?

   a. _____

   b. _____

   c. _____

   d. _____

   e. _____

4. What conditions are necessary for a cell to survive?

   a. _____

   b. _____

   c. _____

5. List the different types of cell adaptation.

   a. _____

   b. _____

   c. _____

   d. _____

   e. _____

   f. _____

6. What are the three different types of gangrene?

   a. _____

   b. _____

   c. _____

7. What criteria are used to determine brain death?

   a. _____

   b. _____

   c. _____

   d. _____

CASE STUDY

Jonathan is a 29-year-old diesel mechanic. Because of the high cost of gasoline, Jonathan has been riding his motorcycle rather than his half-ton pickup back and forth to work in order to save money. The temperature is 95°F so Jonathan decided not to wear his helmet on his way home from work. One mile down the freeway, Jonathan changes lanes and is hit by a car. He sustains a severe head injury. He is transported to the local hospital and admitted to the intensive care unit. Jonathan is unresponsive.

What criteria will be used to determine if Jonathan is brain dead?

_____

_____

_____

_____

_____

_____

_____

_____

_____

_____

Neoplasms

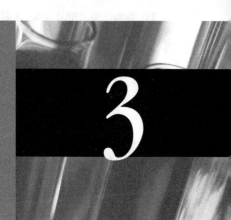

3

COMPLETION

Using the words in the list, complete the following statements:

neoplasm	tumor	leukemia	hematoma
carcinoma	angiogenesis	carcinogens	grading
staging	anaplastic	biopsy	cytology
curative	chemotherapy	preventive	carcinoma in situ

1. _____ determines the degree of abnormality of the neoplasm.

2. A large tumor or swelling filled with blood, commonly called a bruise or contusion, is called a _____.

3. A _____ is a swelling or neoplasm.

4. The largest group of malignant neoplasms is called _____.

5. Cancer-causing agents are known as _____.

6. _____ considers the degree of spread.

7. Removing a small piece of tissue for microscopic examination is known as _____.

8. _____ is the examination of cells.

9. Treatment aimed at a cure is known as _____.

10. Atypical cells that just sit in the epithelial layer of tissue and have not broken through the basement membrane are called _____.

11. New growth of blood vessels is called _____.

12. _____ is the malignant disease of the bone marrow causing an increase in white blood cell production.

13. Reduction in fat intake and an increase in fiber, fruits, and vegetable consumption are examples of _____ measures.

14. _____ is the use of medications to kill or inhibit the growth of neoplasms.

15. The more abnormal the tissue appears in comparison to its normal tissue, the more undifferentiated or _____ it is.

SHORT ANSWER

Answer the following questions:

1. What is a carcinoma?

   _____

   _____

   _____

2. What is a sarcoma?

   _____

   _____

   _____

3. What is a lymphoma?

   _____

   _____

   _____

4. What is a glioma?

   _____

   _____

   _____

5. What is a melanoma?

   _____

   _____

   _____

6. There are several factors that regulate the growth of normal cells. List them.

   a. _____

   b. _____

   c. _____

7. Describe a metastatic neoplasm.

   _____

   _____

   _____

8. What causes genetic mutation?

   a. _____

   b. _____

   c. _____

   d. _____

9. In what ways are hyperplasias and neoplasms similar?

   a. _____

   b. _____

10. In what ways do hyperplasias and neoplasms differ?

    a. _____

    b. _____

    c. _____

    d. _____

    e. _____

11. Describe precancerous or preneoplastic cells.

    _____

    _____

    _____

12. Describe carcinoma in situ.

    _____

    _____

    _____

13. What happens in the final stage of cancer development?

    _____

    _____

    _____

14. How do carcinomas spread?

    _____

    _____

    _____

15. Why are lymph nodes surgically removed?

a. _____

b. _____

16. How does the spread of carcinomas differ from the spread of sarcomas?

a. _____

b. _____

17. List the common sites of bloodstream metastasis.

a. _____

b. _____

c. _____

18. List the chemical carcinomas and what kinds of cancer they cause.

a. _____

b. _____

c. _____

d. _____

19. What effect does estrogen have on prostate cancer?

_____

_____

_____

20. Besides estrogen, what other treatments can be done to slow the growth of prostatic tumors?

_____

_____

_____

21. What types of radioactive materials have the greatest carcinogenic potential?

a. _____

b. _____

c. _____

22. The Epstein-Barr virus has been associated with what type of cancer?

_____

_____

_____

23. What viruses have been associated with the development of cancer?

a. _____

b. _____

c. _____

24. What two types of cancer have a higher incidence in certain families?

a. _____

b. _____

25. List the personal risk behaviors that put an individual at increased risk for developing cancer.

a. _____

b. _____

c. _____

d. _____

26. List the factors that decrease a female's risk for developing breast cancer.

a. _____

b. _____

c. _____

27. Pregnancy and childbirth appears to be a protective mechanism for women from what types of cancer?

a. _____

b. _____

c. _____

28. What cancer-causing behavior is considered the most preventable?

_____

_____

_____

29. Increased consumption of what dietary items is considered preventive in cancer development?

a. _____

b. _____

c. _____

30. What are the American Cancer Society's recommendations for cancer prevention?

a. _____

b. _____

c. _____

d. _____

e. _____

f. _____

g. _____

h. _____

i. _____

j. _____

31. What groups and ages of people are affected by cancer?

_____

_____

_____

32. Excluding the skin, what are the most common sites of cancer?

a. _____

b. _____

c. _____

d. _____

e. _____

33. List common routine cancer screening measures.

a. _____

b. _____

c. _____

d. _____

e. _____

34. What does the acronym CAUTION stand for?

a. C _____

b. A _____

c. U _____

d. T _____

e. I _____

f. O _____

g. N _____

35. What is the most definitive test for diagnosing cancer?

_____

_____

_____

36. List the different methods utilized to obtain a biopsy?

   a. _____

   b. _____

   c. _____

   d. _____

37. List the different signs and symptoms of cancer.

   a. _____

   b. _____

   c. _____

   d. _____

   e. _____

   f. _____

   g. _____

38. What are the three major types of cancer treatment?

   a. _____

   b. _____

   c. _____

39. What are the three possible outcomes from a surgical intervention in the treatment of cancer?

   a. _____

   b. _____

   c. _____

4 Inflammation and Infection

DEFINING TERMS

Define the following terms:

1. bacteria _____

_____

2. trauma _____

_____

3. hyperemia _____

_____

4. sebaceous _____

_____

5. odoriferous _____

_____

6. chemotaxis _____

_____

7. pus _____

_____

8. lesion _____

_____

9. scab _____

_____

10. purulent _____

_____

11. pyogenic _____

_____

12. abscess _____

_____

13. cellulitis _____

_____

14. fistula _____

_____

15. keloid _____

_____

16. ulcer _____

_____

17. infection _____

_____

18. adhesion _____

_____

19. periorbital cellulitis _____

_____

20. empyema _____

_____

SHORT ANSWER

Answer the following questions:

1. What are the body's three basic lines of defense?

a. _____

b. _____

c. _____

2. Describe inflammation.

_____

_____

_____

3. What are the three primary goals of the inflammatory response?

    a. _____

    b. _____

    c. _____

4. When does the inflammatory process occur?

    _____

    _____

    _____

5. What is the function of hyperemia?

    _____

    _____

    _____

6. What are the "foot soldiers" of the inflammatory process?

    _____

    _____

    _____

7. Describe chronic inflammation.

    _____

    _____

    _____

8. What does a microscopic examination of chronic inflammation reveal?

    _____

    _____

    _____

9. What happens if macrophages are unable to overcome the invader and protect the host?

    _____

    _____

    _____

10. What is serous exudate?

    a. _____

    b. _____

    c. _____

11. What is fibrinous exudate?

a. _____

b. _____

c. _____

12. Describe a lesion.

a. _____

b. _____

13. List three inflammatory lesions.

a. _____

b. _____

c. _____

14. What is the typical cause of an abscess?

_____

_____

_____

15. How is an abscess formed?

_____

_____

_____

16. List three examples of an abscess.

a. _____

b. _____

c. _____

17. What are the signs of acute inflammation?

a. _____

b. _____

c. _____

d. _____

18. What is the "head" of an abscess?

a. _____

b. _____

19. What treatment may be necessary to treat a large abscess?

_____

_____

_____

20. What happens when an ulcer is formed?

a. _____

b. _____

21. Where are ulcers commonly found?

a. _____

b. _____

c. _____

22. What is cellulitis?

_____

_____

_____

23. What are the characteristics of cellulitis?

_____

_____

_____

24. What are the causes of cellulitis?

a. _____

b. _____

c. _____

25. How is cellulitis typically treated?

_____

_____

_____

26. What are the two basic methods of tissue repair?

a. _____

b. _____

27. What is the end product of fibrous connective tissue repair?

_____

_____

_____

Immune System Diseases and Disorders

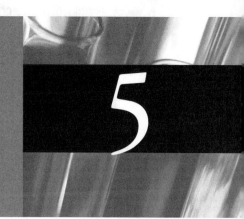

5

MATCHING

Match the following terms with the correct definition:

_____ **1.** autoimmune

_____ **2.** antigen

_____ **3.** hemolytic

_____ **4.** rheumatoid factor

_____ **5.** urticaria

_____ **6.** immunodeficiency

_____ **7.** ptosis

_____ **8.** cytoxic

_____ **9.** anaphylaxis

_____ **10.** diplopia

a. lack of immunity

b. RF

c. double vision

d. allergens

e. drooping eyelids

f. hives

g. severe allergic reaction

h. cell killing

i. blood destroying

j. immunity against self

SHORT ANSWER

Answer the following questions:

1. What are the primary and secondary organs of the immune system?

a. _____

b. _____

c. _____

d. _____

e. _____

f. _____

2. What are the major cells of the immune system?

_____

_____

_____

3. List the cells of the immune system.

a. _____

b. _____

c. _____

d. _____

e. _____

4. What happens to monocytes and macrophages in the presence of pathogens and foreign substances?

_____

_____

_____

5. Where are lymphocytes formed?

_____

_____

_____

6. What do the lymphocytes that remain in the bone marrow become?

_____

_____

_____

7. What happens to the lymphocytes that migrate to the thymus?

_____

_____

_____

8. What is the job of the B lymphocytes?

_____

_____

_____

9. Name two types of immune responses.

a. _____

b. _____

38. What is the treatment for an anaphylactic reaction?

a. _____

b. _____

c. _____

d. _____

e. _____

39. How are food allergies often diagnosed?

_____

_____

_____

40. What are the symptoms of food allergies?

a. _____

b. _____

c. _____

41. What allergens are common causes of contact dermatitis?

a. _____

b. _____

c. _____

d. _____

e. _____

f. _____

g. _____

42. What are autoimmune disorders?

_____

_____

_____

43. List some examples of autoimmune disorders.

a. _____

b. _____

c. _____

d. _____

e. _____

44. What is the cause of rheumatic fever?

_____

_____

_____

45. What are the symptoms of rheumatic fever?

a. _____

b. _____

c. _____

46. What is the best preventive measure against rheumatic fever?

_____

_____

_____

47. What does rheumatoid arthritis cause?

_____

_____

_____

48. With what is the cause of rheumatoid arthritis associated?

_____

_____

_____

49. What is found in the blood that is indicative of rheumatoid arthritis?

_____

_____

_____

50. Describe the progression of rheumatoid arthritis.

_____

_____

_____

51. What is another name for rheumatoid arthritis?

_____

_____

_____

52. What is the treatment for rheumatoid arthritis?

a. _____

b. _____

c. _____

d. _____

53. What is a characteristic of myasthenia gravis?

_____

_____

_____

54. What does myasthenia gravis affect?

_____

_____

_____

55. What are the symptoms of myasthenia gravis?

a. _____

b. _____

c. _____

d. _____

e. _____

f. _____

56. What is the treatment for myasthenia gravis?

a. _____

b. _____

c. _____

57. What problem will cause death in the person with myasthenia gravis?

_____

_____

_____

58. What is the cause of Type 1 diabetes mellitus?

_____

_____

_____

59. What common viral infections lead to diabetes?

a. _____

b. _____

c. _____

60. List the two types of lupus erythematosus.

a. _____

b. _____

61. What is the classic sign of lupus erythematosus?

_____

_____

_____

62. List the other symptoms of lupus erythematosus.

a. _____

b. _____

c. _____

d. _____

63. What is the treatment for lupus erythematosus?

a. _____

b. _____

c. _____

64. What is scleroderma?

_____

_____

_____

65. What is the treatment of scleroderma?

a. _____

b. _____

c. _____

d. _____

66. What happens when antibodies react with antigens?

_____

_____

_____

67. What are the symptoms of a transfusion reaction?

   a. _____

   b. _____

   c. _____

68. Describe erythroblastosis fetalis.

   _____

   _____

   _____

69. What is the treatment for erythroblastosis fetalis?

   _____

   _____

   _____

70. When does chronic organ rejection occur?

   _____

   _____

   _____

71. What is an immunodeficiency disorder?

   _____

   _____

   _____

72. How is immune deficiency acquired?

   a. _____

   b. _____

   c. _____

73. What disorders commonly lead to immunodeficiency?

   a. _____

   b. _____

   c. _____

   d. _____

74. What does acquired immunodeficiency syndrome cause?

   _____

   _____

   _____

75. What is the causative organism of AIDS?

_____

_____

_____

76. List the four stages of HIV.

a. _____

b. _____

c. _____

d. _____

77. How is HIV transmitted?

a. _____

b. _____

78. List the three primary ways HIV can be spread or transmitted.

a. _____

b. _____

c. _____

Musculoskeletal System Diseases and Disorders

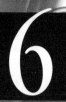

6

COMPLETION

Using the words in the list, complete the following statements:

tophi   interphalangeal   anaerobic   myelogram
rickets   kyphosis   lordosis   scoliosis
densitometry   compression   flexion   abduction
dowager's hump   adduction   rotation   circumduction
elevation   electromyography   nondisplaced   striated
osteomalacia   extension

1. Circular movement is known as _____.

2. Muscle that looks like stripes or bands is _____.

3. _____ is osteomalacia in children.

4. Small whitish nodules are called _____.

5. Bending is also called _____.

6. Humpback is known medically as _____.

7. The measurement of bone thickness is called _____.

8. Lateral curve of the spine is called _____.

9. Moving a body part toward the body's midline is called _____.

10. When you reach out, you are experiencing _____.

11. Turning on the axis is called _____.

12. _____ is when a bone is smashed down on itself.

13. Lifting is also called _____.

14. _____ _____ is abnormal curvature in the upper thoracic spine.

15. A fracture that is not out of alignment is said to be _____.

16. _____ is also called swayback.

17. EMG is the abbreviation for _____.

18. _____ means "without air."

19. _____ means "between finger bones."

20. Special X-rays after the injection of dye into the spinal cord to reveal compression of the spinal cord or spinal nerves is called a _____.

MATCHING

Match the following terms with the correct definition:

_____ 1. transverse

_____ 2. oblique

_____ 3. spiral

_____ 4. stellate

_____ 5. intertrochanteric

a. star-like pattern
b. runs across at a 90-degree angle
c. twisted around the bone
d. within the trochanter of the femur
e. run in a transverse pattern

MATCHING

Match the following terms with the correct definition:

_____ 1. open fracture

_____ 2. simple fracture

_____ 3. comminuted

_____ 4. stress fracture

_____ 5. greenstick

a. more than two ends or fragments
b. bone is protruding through the skin
c. incomplete fracture
d. no opening in the skin
e. too much weight-bearing or pressure

30. What are the symptoms of osteomyelitis?

    a. _____

    b. _____

    c. _____

    d. _____

    e. _____

31. What is the treatment for osteomyelitis?

    a. _____

    b. _____

32. What is osteomalacia?

    _____

    _____

    _____

33. What is the cause of osteomalacia?

    _____

    _____

    _____

34. What are the symptoms of osteomalacia?

    a. _____

    b. _____

    c. _____

35. What is arthritis?

    _____

    _____

    _____

36. What are the two groups of arthritis?

    a. _____

    b. _____

37. What is the most common type of arthritis?

    _____

    _____

    _____

38. What is rheumatoid arthritis?

_____

_____

_____

39. What is another name for osteoarthritis?

_____

_____

_____

40. What is osteoarthritis?

_____

_____

_____

41. Which joints are most frequently affected in osteoarthritis?

a. _____

b. _____

c. _____

d. _____

42. What are the risk factors for developing osteoarthritis?

a. _____

b. _____

c. _____

d. _____

e. _____

43. What is the treatment for osteoarthritis?

a. _____

b. _____

c. _____

d. _____

e. _____

f. _____

g. _____

44. What is rheumatoid arthritis?

_____

_____

_____

45. What is gout?

_____

_____

_____

46. Which joint is affected most often in gout?

_____

_____

_____

47. What are the symptoms of gout?

a. _____

b. _____

c. _____

d. _____

48. Which sex is most frequently affected in gout?

_____

_____

_____

49. What is the treatment for gout?

a. _____

b. _____

c. _____

50. What is hallux valgus?

_____

_____

_____

51. What is another name for hallux valgus?

_____

_____

_____

52. Which sex is most frequently affected with hallux valgus?

_____

_____

_____

53. What are the causes of hallux valgus?

a. _____

b. _____

54. What are the symptoms of hallux valgus?

a. _____

b. _____

c. _____

55. How is hallux valgus treated?

a. _____

b. _____

c. _____

d. _____

56. What are the classic signs of temporomandibular joint syndrome (TMJ)?

a. _____

b. _____

57. What are the causes of TMJ?

a. _____

b. _____

c. _____

d. _____

58. What is the most common type of muscular dystrophy?

_____

_____

_____

59. Who is most frequently affected by Duchenne's muscular dystrophy?

_____

_____

_____

60. Which sex is most frequently affected by Duchenne's muscular dystrophy?

_____

_____

_____

61. What is a ganglion cyst?

_____

_____

_____

62. What is the cause of a ganglion cyst?

_____

_____

_____

63. How is a ganglion cyst treated?

a. _____

b._____

64. What is tetanus?

_____

_____

_____

65. What are the characteristics of tetanus?

_____

_____

_____

66. What is the causative organism for tetanus?

_____

_____

_____

67. Where is _Clostridium tetani_ found?

_____

_____

_____

68. What muscles are affected most often in tetanus?

_____

_____

_____

69. What are the symptoms of tetanus?

a. _____

b._____

    c. _____

    d. _____

    e. _____

    f. _____

70. How is tetanus treated?

    a. _____

    b. _____

71. What does tetanus toxoid do?

_____

_____

_____

72. What type of care is needed for the patient with tetanus?

    a. _____

    b. _____

73. What is the most common neoplasm of the musculoskeletal system?

_____

_____

_____

74. What is the most common marrow tumor?

_____

_____

_____

75. What are the primary tumors of the bone marrow?

    a. _____

    b. _____

76. What are the most common symptoms of the musculoskeletal system?

    a. _____

    b. _____

77. What diagnostic tests are performed to confirm the diagnosis for neoplasms of the musculoskeletal system?

    a. _____

    b. _____

    c. _____

    d. _____

78. What treatments are used for malignant tumors of the musculoskeletal system?

a. _____

b. _____

c. _____

79. What is the prognosis for malignant neoplasms of the musculoskeletal system?

_____

_____

_____

80. What is the main cause of musculoskeletal problems in the United States?

_____

_____

_____

81. What is the most common injury to the bone?

_____

_____

_____

82. What chronic disorder is among the top 10 reasons for seeking medical attention?

_____

_____

_____

83. What musculoskeletal disorders are among the top 10 reasons why people seek medical treatment?

_____

_____

_____

84. What is a fracture?

a. _____

b. _____

85. What are the causes of fractures?

a. _____

b. _____

86. Describe the following fractures:

a. open _____

b. closed or simple _____

   c. greenstick   _____

   d. displaced   _____

   e. nondisplaced   _____

   f. comminuted   _____

   g. compression   _____

   h. impacted   _____

   i. avulsion   _____

   j. longitudinal   _____

   k. transverse   _____

   l. oblique   _____

   m. spiral   _____

   n. stellate   _____

   o. intracapsular   _____

   p. extracapsular   _____

   q. intertrochanteric   _____

   r. femoral neck/subcapital   _____

87. How are fractures treated?

   a. _____

   b. _____

   c. _____

   d. _____

   e. _____

88. Describe a closed reduction.

_____

_____

_____

89. How long does it take for fractures to heal?

_____

_____

_____

90. What is the benefit of traction when treating fractures?

   a. _____

   b. _____

   c. _____

91. What are two types of traction?

    a. _____

    b. _____

92. What are the complications of fractures?

    a. _____

    b. _____

    c. _____

    d. _____

93. What is a strain?

_____

_____

_____

94. What are the symptoms of a strain?

    a. _____

    b. _____

    c. _____

95. What is the treatment of a strain?

    a. _____

    b. _____

    c. _____

    d. _____

96. What is a sprain?

_____

_____

_____

97. What are the symptoms of a sprain?

    a. _____

    b. _____

    c. _____

    d. _____

98. What does the acronym RICE mean?

    R _____

    I _____

    C _____

    E _____

99. In the case of a joint dislocation, why would general anesthesia be necessary?

a. _____

b. _____

100. What disorders that affect the spine also lead to low back pain?

a. _____

b. _____

c. _____

d. _____

e. _____

101. What is the treatment for low back pain?

a. _____

b. _____

c. _____

d. _____

102. What is a herniated disk?

_____

_____

_____

103. What is sciatica?

_____

_____

_____

104. What diagnostic tests are performed to confirm of the diagnosis of a herniated disk?

a. _____

b. _____

c. _____

105. How is a slipped disk treated?

a. _____

b. _____

c. _____

106. What is bursitis?

_____

_____

_____

107. What is the job of the bursa?

_____

_____

_____

108. What are the symptoms of bursitis?

_____

_____

_____

109. What is the treatment for bursitis?

a. _____

b. _____

c. _____

d. _____

110. What is tennis elbow?

_____

_____

_____

111. How is tennis elbow diagnosed?

_____

_____

_____

112. What is tendonitis?

_____

_____

_____

113. What area of the body is most often affected by tendonitis?

_____

_____

_____

114. What is the treatment for tendonitis?

a. _____

b. _____

c. _____

d. _____

e. _____

f. _____

115. Describe carpal tunnel syndrome (CTS).

_____

_____

_____

116. What are the symptoms of CTS?

a. _____

b. _____

c. _____

d. _____

e. _____

117. How is CTS treated?

a. _____

b. _____

c. _____

d. _____

e. _____

f. _____

118. How can CTS be prevented?

a. _____

b. _____

c. _____

119. What is plantar fasciitis also called?

a. _____

b. _____

120. What are the common symptoms of plantar fasciitis?

_____

_____

_____

121. How is plantar fasciitis treated?

a. _____

b. _____

c. _____

d. _____

e. _____

f. _____

122. What is the rotator cuff?

_____

_____

_____

123. What are the common causes of tears in the rotator cuff?

_____

_____

_____

124. How is a torn rotator cuff diagnosed?

a. _____

b. _____

c. _____

125. How is a rotator cuff treated?

_____

_____

_____

126. What is the postoperative treatment for a torn rotator cuff?

a. _____

b. _____

c. _____

d. _____

127. What is the cause of a torn meniscus?

_____

_____

_____

128. What are the symptoms of a torn meniscus?

a. _____

b. _____

c. _____

129. What is the treatment for a torn meniscus?

a. _____

b. _____

c. _____

d. _____

e. _____

130. How do cruciate ligament tears occur?

_____

_____

_____

131. What is the treatment for a cruciate ligament injury?

a. _____

b. _____

132. What are shin splints?

_____

_____

_____

133. What are the common symptoms of shin splints?

_____

_____

_____

134. What is the treatment for shin splints?

a. _____

b. _____

c. _____

d. _____

135. What is de Quervain's disease?

_____

_____

_____

136. What are the symptoms of de Quervain's disease?

a. _____

b. _____

137. How does tuberculosis affect the bone?

_____

_____

_____

138. How is tuberculosis of the bone treated?

_____

_____

_____

139. What are the symptoms of Paget's disease?

a. _____

b. _____

c. _____

140. What is the treatment for Paget's disease?

_____

_____

_____

141. What happens to the musculoskeletal system as an individual ages?

a. _____

b. _____

c. _____

d. _____

e. _____

f. _____

7 Blood and Blood-Forming Organs Diseases and Disorders

DEFINING TERMS

Define the following terms:

1. erythrocytopenia _____

   _____

2. erythrocytosis _____

   _____

3. leukocytopenia _____

   _____

4. leukocytosis _____

   _____

5. thrombocytopenia _____

   _____

6. thrombocytosis _____

   _____

7. petechiae _____

   _____

8. ecchymosis _____

   _____

9. epistaxis _____

   _____

10. hemolyzed _____

    _____

11. syncope _____

_____

12. dyspnea _____

_____

13. tachycardia _____

_____

14. tachypnea _____

_____

15. hemarthrosis _____

_____

16. purpura _____

_____

MATCHING

Match the disease condition with the correct definition.

_____ 1. anemia

_____ 2. pernicious anemia

_____ 3. hemolytic anemia

_____ 4. sickle cell anemia

_____ 5. hemorrhagic anemia

_____ 6. aplastic anemia

_____ 7. pancytopenia

_____ 8. mononucleosis

_____ 9. leukemia

_____ 10. lymphoma

a. neoplasms of lymphoid tissue

b. defense mechanism against malaria

c. abnormally high number of immature leukocytes

d. lack of intrinsic factor

e. "kissing disease"

f. decrease in the oxygen-carrying ability of the red blood cell

g. failure of bone marrow to produce blood components

h. increased destruction of red blood cells

i. acute loss of large amounts of blood

SHORT ANSWER

Answer the following questions:

1. What is the major function of the blood?

_____

_____

_____

2. What is the role of leukocytes?

_____

_____

_____

3. Describe plasma.

_____

_____

_____

4. What color is venous blood?

_____

_____

_____

5. How much blood is circulating in the body of an adult?

_____

_____

_____

6. What is the pH of blood?

_____

_____

_____

7. What is the function of erythrocytes?

_____

_____

_____

8. What is a normal erythrocyte count?

_____

_____

_____

9. What is the life span of an erythrocyte?

_____

_____

_____

10. Where are erythrocytes produced?

_____

_____

_____

11. What happens to worn-out red blood cells?

a. _____

b. _____

12. What is the function of hemoglobin?

_____

_____

_____

13. What is the normal range for the hemoglobin of an adult female and male?

a. female: _____

b. male: _____

14. What is the function of leukocytes?

_____

_____

_____

15. What is the normal range for white blood cells?

_____

_____

_____

16. What is the indication of a white blood cell count greater than 11,000?

_____

_____

_____

17. What is another name for platelets?

_____

_____

_____

18. What is the average number of platelets for an adult?

_____

_____

19. Describe the composition of plasma.

_____

_____

_____

20. List the phases of blood coagulation.

a. _____

b. _____

c. _____

d. _____

21. List the four types of blood.

a. _____

b. _____

c. _____

d. _____

22. What is the difference between Rh negative blood and Rh positive blood?

_____

_____

_____

23. List the blood-forming organs.

a. _____

b. _____

c. _____

d. _____

24. What are the symptoms of anemia?

a. _____

b. _____

c. _____

d. _____

e. _____

25. What are the common symptoms of erythrocytosis?

a. _____

b. _____

c. _____

d. _____

e. _____

26. What happens when an individual has leukocytopenia?

_____

_____

_____

27. What effect does leukocytosis have on the body?

a. _____

b. _____

28. What are the symptoms of thrombocytopenia?

a. _____

b. _____

c. _____

d. _____

29. What complication results from having thrombocytopenia?

_____

_____

_____

30. What does the abbreviation CBC stand for? What tests are performed when a CBC is ordered?

_____

_____

_____

31. What is the hematocrit?

_____

_____

_____

32. What is the hemoglobin?

_____

_____

_____

33. What is a bleeding time?

_____

_____

_____

34. What do the abbreviations PT and PTT stand for? What do these tests measure?

_____

_____

_____

35. What other tests are used to diagnose diseases and disorders of the blood-forming organs?

a. _____

b. _____

36. What is anemia?

a. _____

b. _____

37. What disorders or diseases may lead to anemia?

a. _____

b. _____

c. _____

38. What are the common symptoms of anemia?

a. _____

b. _____

c. _____

d. _____

e. _____

f. _____

g. _____

h. _____

i. _____

39. What are the causes of iron deficiency anemia?

a. _____

b. _____

40. What are the causes of folic acid deficiency anemia?

a. _____

b. _____

c. _____

d. _____

41. What is pernicious anemia?

_____

_____

_____

42. How is pernicious anemia treated?

_____

_____

_____

43. What is the characteristic of hemolytic anemia?

_____

_____

_____

44. What is the treatment for hemolytic anemia?

a. _____

b. _____

45. What ethnic group is affected by sickle cell anemia?

_____

_____

_____

46. What is the theory to explain the development of sickle cell anemia?

_____

_____

_____

47. Acute loss of large amounts of blood leads to what type of anemia?

_____

_____

_____

48. What is the treatment of choice for hemorrhagic anemia?

_____

_____

_____

49. What is the characteristic of aplastic anemia?

_____

_____

_____

50. What is pancytopenia?

_____

_____

_____

51. What are the causes of aplastic anemia?

a. _____

b. _____

c. _____

d. _____

52. What are possible treatments for aplastic anemia?

a. _____

b. _____

c. _____

53. List two other names for polycythemia.

a. _____

b. _____

54. What is the cause of polycythemia?

_____

_____

_____

55. What is the treatment for polycythemia?

_____

_____

_____

56. What are the symptoms of mononucleosis?

a. _____

b. _____

c. _____

57. What is the treatment for mononucleosis?

a. _____

b. _____

c. _____

58. What is another name for mononucleosis?

_____

_____

_____

59. What is leukemia?

_____

_____

_____

60. What are the characteristics of leukemia?

a. _____

b. _____

61. What are the symptoms of leukemia?

a. _____

b. _____

c. _____

d. _____

e. _____

f. _____

g. _____

62. What is the treatment for leukemia?

a. _____

b. _____

c. _____

63. What is lymphoma?

_____

_____

_____

64. What is Hodgkin's disease?

_____

_____

_____

65. What are the characteristics of Hodgkin's disease?

a. _____

b. _____

c. _____

66. What is the cause of Hodgkin's disease?

_____

_____

_____

67. How is Hodgkin's disease diagnosed?

a. _____

b. _____

68. How is Hodgkin's disease treated?

a. _____

b. _____

69. What is non-Hodgkin's lymphoma?

_____

_____

_____

70. What are the symptoms of non-Hodgkin's disease?

a. _____

b. _____

c. _____

d. _____

71. What is the treatment for non-Hodgkin's lymphoma?

_____

_____

_____

72. What is multiple myeloma?

_____

_____

_____

73. How is the diagnosis of multiple myeloma confirmed?

a. _____

b. _____

c. _____

d. _____

74. What is hemophilia?

_____

_____

_____

75. What are the symptoms of hemophilia?

a. _____

b. _____

c. _____

76. What is the treatment for hemophilia?

a. _____

b. _____

c. _____

77. What is thrombocytopenia?

_____

_____

_____

78. What are the characteristics of thrombocytopenia?

a. _____

b. _____

c. _____

d. _____

e. _____

f. _____

79. How is thrombocytopenia diagnosed?

a. _____

b. _____

c. _____

80. How is thrombocytopenia treated?

a. _____

b. _____

c. _____

d. _____

81. What is disseminated intravascular coagulation?

_____

_____

_____

82. When does disseminated intravascular coagulation occur?

_____

_____

_____

83. What are the symptoms of disseminated intravascular coagulation?

a. _____

b. _____

c. _____

d. _____

e. _____

84. What is the treatment for disseminated intravascular coagulation?

a. _____

b. _____

85. What is thalassemia?

_____

_____

_____

86. What is another name for von Willebrand's disease?

_____

_____

_____

87. What is the cause of von Willebrand's disease?

_____

_____

_____

88. What is the most common disorder of the blood in the older adult?

_____

_____

_____

Cardiovascular System Diseases and Disorders

8

COMPLETION

Using the words in the list, complete the following statements:

plaque	cyanosis	diastolic	chest pain
palpitations	dyspnea	embolus	murmur
fibrillation	ischemia	patency	systolic
tachycardia	thrombus	hypotension	hypertension
cardiac arrest	arrhythmia	auscultation	bradycardia
hemorrhage	blood pressure		

1. The top or first recorded number in the blood pressure, caused by the contraction of the ventricle is the _____ blood pressure.

2. Difficult breathing is also known as _____.

3. _____ _____ is the level of pressure of the blood pushing against the walls of the vessels as it is delivered throughout the body.

4. Another word for _____ is openness.

5. A blood pressure greater than 140/90 is considered _____.

6. Blood vessels containing fatty, cholesterol deposits are called

   _____.

7. A blood clot that breaks loose and floats in the blood, possibly occluding or stopping blood flow is known as a(n) _____.

8. _____ is death of organs due to lack of blood supply.

9. An irregular heart rhythm is called a(n) _____.

10. A wild, uncontrolled arrhythmia is called a(n) _____.

11. _____ is abnormal blood loss.

12. Another word for rapid heart rate is _____.

13. Abnormal heart rate that the individual can feel or is very aware of is called _____.

14. _____ is a slow heart rate.

15. The bottom number or lower number in the blood pressure is known as the _____ blood pressure.

DEFINING ABBREVIATIONS

Define the following abbreviations:

1. CVA _____

2. AV node _____

3. MI _____

4. EKG or ECG _____

5. BP _____

6. PVD _____

7. CHF _____

8. CAD _____

9. CABG _____

10. CPR _____

11. TPA _____

12. RHD _____

13. DVT _____

14. hgb _____

15. hct _____

MATCHING

Match the following diagnostic terms with the correct definition:

_____ **1.** EKG

_____ **2.** hemoglobin

_____ **3.** arteriogram

_____ **4.** ultrasound

_____ **5.** angiogram

_____ **6.** CPK, LDH

_____ **7.** Doppler

_____ **8.** TPA

_____ **9.** prothrombin time

_____ **10.** cardiac catheterization

a. invasive procedure used to sample the blood in the chambers of the heart to determine the oxygen content

b. X-ray of a vessel

c. blood tests that measure the levels of enzymes that help determine the severity and time of the heart attack

d. use of sound waves for diagnostic purposes

e. a device used for listening to the heart and movement of blood in vessels

f. carries the oxygen in the blood

g. graph of the electrical activity of the heart

h. X-ray of an artery

i. "clot buster"

j. blood test to monitor the anticoagulant drug level

SHORT ANSWER

Describe the following surgical procedures and when they are indicated:

1. Coronary artery bypass graft

_____

_____

_____

2. Endarterectomy

_____

_____

_____

3. Angioplasty

_____

_____

_____

4. Vein stripping

_____

_____

_____

5. Embolectomy/thrombectomy

_____

_____

_____

SHORT ANSWER

For each of the cardiovascular diseases, describe the condition, then list the symptoms and tell how the disease is diagnosed.

1. Aneurysm

_____

_____

_____

2. Arteriosclerosis/atherosclerosis

_____

_____

_____

3. Cerebrovascular accident

_____

_____

_____

4. Coronary artery disease

_____

_____

_____

5. Deep vein thrombosis

_____

_____

_____

MATCHING

Match the disease with the correct definition.

_____ **1.** hay fever

_____ **2.** pharyngitis

_____ **3.** chronic bronchitis

_____ **4.** pulmonary abscess

_____ **5.** tuberculosis

_____ **6.** adult respiratory distress syndrome

_____ **7.** pleural effusion

_____ **8.** coccidioidomycosis

_____ **9.** Legionnaire's disease

_____ **10.** laryngitis

a. sore throat

b. "shock lung"

c. Legionnaire's lung

d. hydrothorax

e. allergic rhinitis

f. "desert fever"

g. "consumption"

h. "smoker's cough"

i. lung abscess

j. hoarseness

DEFINING TERMS

Define the following terms:

1. analgesic _____

_____

2. antipyretic _____

_____

3. apnea _____

_____

4. bronchiectasis _____

_____

5. clubbing _____

_____

6. cyanosis _____

_____

7. dyspnea   _____

_____

8. hypoxia   _____

_____

9. orthopnea   _____

_____

10. productive cough   _____

_____

11. rales   _____

_____

12. rhinorrhea   _____

_____

13. rhonchi   _____

_____

14. sputum   _____

_____

15. tachypnea   _____

_____

16. thoracentesis   _____

_____

17. wheezing   _____

_____

18. atelectasis   _____

_____

19. hemoptysis   _____

_____

20. alveoli   _____

_____

SHORT ANSWER

Answer the following questions.

1. Describe mechanical ventilation:

_____

_____

_____

2. Describe influenza immunization.

_____

_____

_____

3. Describe surgical resection.

_____

_____

_____

4. Describe thoracentesis.

_____

_____

_____

5. Describe salt-water gargles.

_____

_____

_____

CONDITION TABLE

Complete the following table:

Condition and Definition	Symptoms	How Diagnosed	Treatment
Common Cold			

(continued)

CONDITION TABLE (continued)

Condition and Definition	Symptoms	How Diagnosed	Treatment
Hay Fever			
Sinusitis			
Pharyngitis			
Acute Bronchitis			
Influenza			
Chronic Obstructive Lung Disease			
Pneumonia			

CONDITION TABLE (continued)

Condition and Definition	Symptoms	How Diagnosed	Treatment
Tuberculosis			
Pleurisy			
Pulmonary Embolism			
Legionnaire's Disease			
Pneumothorax			

COMPLETION

Complete the following statements:

1. _____ is when the individual is unable to breathe unless the individual is in a sitting position.

2. Musical sounds when listening to the lungs is called _____.

3. A runny nose is also called _____.

4. The medical term for low oxygen in the blood is _____.

5. The medical term for coughing up blood is _____.

6. Bad, painful, or difficult breathing is called _____.

7. Medications used to reduce fevers are called _____.

8. Absence of respirations is known as _____.

9. _____ is poor distal circulation and oxgenation.

10. Pain relievers are called _____.

11. A bluish color to the skin is called _____.

12. Rapid breathing is known as _____.

13. Dry, rattling sounds when listening to the lungs is called _____.

14. The surgical puncture of the thorax is known as _____.

15. _____ is fluids or secretions coughed up from the lungs.

16. _____ is high-pitched whistling sounds caused by partial obstruction of the lungs.

17. The grape-like clusters of air sacs at the distal end of the terminal bronchioles are known as _____.

18. A(n) _____ _____ is one in which there is sputum of excessive mucus.

19. The visual examination of the bronchi is called _____.

20. Removing tissue for examination under the microscope is known as a(n) _____.

21. Allergic rhinitis is commonly known as _____.

22. _____ is inflammation of the mucous membrane lining of the sinuses.

23. Pharyngitis is commonly known as a(n) _____ _____.

24. Inflammation of the vocal cords and larynx is called _____.

25. A highly contagious respiratory infection characterized by sudden onset of fever, chills, headache, and back pain is called _____.

26. A group of diseases characterized by the inability to get air in and out of the lungs is known as _____ _____

_____ _____.

27. Collapse or airless state of part or all of the lung is called _____.

28. Inflammation of the lung is called _____.

29. _____ was formerly called consumption.

30. _____ _____ is the leading cause of cancer deaths in the United States.

31. Inflammation of the membranes covering the lung is called _____.

32. Collection of air in the pleural space is called _____.

33. _____ is a procedure done in order to withdraw air and insert a chest tube to assist in reexpanding the lung.

34. A collection of fluid in the chest is known as _____.

35. A clot that commonly develops in the legs, breaks off, and gets stuck in the pulmonary artery is called a(n) _____ _____.

36. _____ is an example of a fungal disease of the lung.

37. _____ _____ is the most preventable risk factor for developing lung cancer.

38. The type of infection that accounts for approximately 80 percent of all infections is called _____ _____.

39. The most common cause for lost days of work for adults is _____ _____ _____.

40. The name of the virus responsible for upper respiratory infections is _____.

10 Lymphatic System Diseases and Disorders

DEFINING TERMS

Define the following terms:

1. lymph _____

2. lymphocytes _____

3. lymphocytosis _____

4. lymphocytopenia _____

5. lymphangiography _____

6. lymphadenopathy _____

7. lymphangiopathy _____

8. lymphadenitis _____

9. lymphangitis _____

10. lymphedema _____

DEFINING WORD FORMS

Define the following word forms:

1. lymph _____

2. angio _____

3. adeno _____

4. opathy _____

5. graphy _____

6. itis _____

7. edema _____

8. cyto _____

9. osis _____

10. penia _____

SHORT ANSWER

Answer the following questions:

1. List the components of the lymph system.

    _____

    _____

    _____

2. What is the goal of the lymphatic system?

    _____

    _____

    _____

3. What is the job of the lymphatic system?

    _____

    _____

    _____

4. List the common signs and symptoms of the lymphatic system.

a. _____

b. _____

c. _____

d. _____

5. What diagnostic tests are performed in order to confirm a diagnosis of the lymph system?

a. _____

b. _____

c. _____

d. _____

e. _____

f. _____

CONDITION TABLE

Complete the following table:

Condition and Definition	Symptoms	Diagnostic Tests	Treatment Plan
Lymphoma			
Kawasaki Disease			
Lymphedema			
Lymphadenitis			

COMPLETION

Complete the following statements:

1. Inflammation of the lymph gland and/or nodes is known as _____.

2. Neoplasms that affect lymphoid tissue are called _____.

3. _____ is fluid of the lymph system.

4. White blood cells created in the lymphatic system are called _____.

5. Inflammation of the lymph glands is called _____.

6. X-ray of the lymph vessels is called _____.

7. A collection of lymph fluid usually in the extremities is called _____.

8. Disease of the lymph vessels is called _____.

9. _____ _____ is also called mucocutaneous lymph node syndrome.

10. _____ is also called the "kissing disease."

11. Decreased lymphocytes is known medically as _____.

12. Increased lymphocytes are medically called _____.

13. Disease of the lymph glands is called _____.

14. The _____ _____ cell confirms the diagnosis of Hodgkin's disease.

15. The lymphatic system includes the _____, _____, and _____.

11 Digestive System Diseases and Disorders

MATCHING

Match the abbreviation with the correct definition.

_____ **1.** NPO

_____ **2.** UGI

_____ **3.** EGD

_____ **4.** O&P

_____ **5.** IBD

_____ **6.** IBS

a. esophagoduodenoscopy

b. nothing by mouth

c. upper gastrointestinal

d. irritable bowel syndrome

e. ova and parasites

f. inflammatory bowel syndrome

MATCHING

Match the disease with the correct definition.

_____ **1.** gastroenteritis

_____ **2.** Crohn's disease

_____ **3.** inguinal hernia

_____ **4.** irritable bowel syndrome

_____ **5.** hemorrhoids

_____ **6.** gastritis

_____ **7.** dental caries

_____ **8.** gingivitis

_____ **9.** reflux esophagitis

_____ **10.** appendicitis

a. inflammation of the gums with painful bleeding

b. most common intestinal disorder

c. varicose veins in the rectum

d. inflammation of the appendix

e. regional enteritis

f. outpouching of the small intestine and peritoneum into the groin area

g. cavities

h. inflammation of tissue at the lower end of the esophagus

i. inflammation of the stomach

j. inflammation of the stomach and intestine

DEFINING TERMS

Define the following terms:

1. hematochezia _____
   _____

2. diarrhea _____
   _____

3. jejunum _____
   _____

4. achlorhydria _____
   _____

5. defecate _____
   _____

6. epigastric _____
   _____

7. vermiform _____
   _____

8. ileus _____
   _____

9. diverticula _____
   _____

10. asymptomatic _____
    _____

11. melena _____
    _____

12. peritonitis _____
    _____

13. peristalsis _____
    _____

14. intrinsic factor _____
    _____

15. hematemesis _____

_____

16. perforation _____

_____

17. occult _____

_____

18. dental plaque _____

_____

19. malaise _____

_____

20. adhesions _____

_____

DEFINING DIAGNOSTIC TESTS

Define the following diagnostic tests:

1. colonoscopy _____

_____

2. sigmoidoscopy _____

_____

3. occult blood _____

_____

4. ova and parasites _____

_____

5. upper GI series _____

_____

6. barium enema _____

_____

7. gastroscopy _____

_____

8. esophagogastroduodenoscopy _____

_____

9. stool culture _____

_____

10. biopsy _____

_____

CONDITION TABLE

Complete the following table:

Condition and Definition	Symptoms	Diagnosetic Tests	Treatment Plan
Appendicitis			
Reflux Esophagitis			
Pharyngitis			
Crohn's Disease			
Esophageal Varices			
Gastritis			

(continued)

CONDITION TABLE (continued)

Condition and Definition	Symptoms	Diagnosetic Tests	Treatment Plan
Peptic Ulcer			
Dysentery			
Colorectal Cancer			
Hemorrhoids			
Hernias Inguinal			
Diverticulitis/ Diverticulosis			
Gastroenteritis			

COMPLETION

Complete the following statements:

1. The three sections of the small intestine are the _____,

    _____, and _____.

2. Movement of food from the pharynx to the stomach is called _____.

3. The first section of the colon is called the _____.

4. The three parts of the stomach are the _____,

    _____, and _____.

5. The substance necessary for the absorption of vitamin B_{12} is called the

    _____ _____.

6. The condition caused by hard, dry stool is called _____.

7. Loose, watery stools are called _____.

8. The procedure allowing a physician to look directly into the digestive organs is called

    _____.

9. The main reason for tooth loss is _____

    _____.

10. Inflammation of the gums is called _____.

11. The common name for pharyngitis is _____

    _____.

12. The backflow of stomach acids through the cardiac sphincter upward into the esophagus

    is called _____ _____.

13. A _____ _____ is the sliding of part of the

    stomach into the chest cavity.

14. _____ _____ are enlargement of the veins of

    the esophagus.

15. Inflammation of the stomach is called _____.

16. _____ _____ is the result of the loss of

    intrinsic factor.

17. Absence of symptoms is also known as _____.

18. _____ is dark, tarry stools.

19. The absence of hydrochloric acid is called _____.

20. Absence of peristalsis is called _____.

21. Varicose veins of the rectum are called _____.

22. Parts of the intestine that are herniated and become twisted, thus cutting off the blood supply to the organ is called a _____ _____.

23. Inflammatory bowel syndrome is also called _____

     _____.

24. The inflammation of the diverticula is called _____.

25. The condition that causes an individual to be sensitive to gluten proteins is called

     _____ _____.

CASE STUDY

Sue is a 36-year-old registered nurse who has been experiencing pain in the epigastric area after eating spicy foods. She has been complaining of the symptoms for the past few weeks. What disease might she be diagnosed with? How would the diagnosis be made and how would it be treated?

_____

_____

_____

_____

_____

_____

_____

11. Enlargement of the liver is called _____.

12. Self-digestion is known medically as _____.

13. X-ray of the vessels of the gallbladder is called _____.

14. Liver function tests include _____, _____,

    and _____.

15. The use of sound waves to break stones is called _____.

CASE STUDY

Jean is 45 years old and 50 pounds over-weight. For the past 3 weeks, Jean has been experiencing severe right upper gastric pain after eating. What disease might Jean have? What predisposing factors does she have? What symptoms does she have to support your diagnosis? How would your diagnosis be confirmed? What treatment would be done?

_____

_____

_____

_____

_____

_____

_____

13 Urinary System Diseases and Disorders

COMPLETION

Using the words in the list, complete the following statements:

hematuria	pyuria	dysuria	nocturia	oliguria
frequency	urgency	incontinence	pyretic	renal calculi
cystoscopy	cystitis	anuria		

1. Inflammation of the bladder is called _____.

2. Another term for fever is _____.

3. Kidney stones are also called _____ _____.

4. _____ is blood in the urine.

5. The need to urinate "right now" is called _____.

6. _____ is loss of control of urine.

7. The need to urinate at night is called _____.

8. Bad, painful, or difficult urination is called _____.

9. Scant urine production is called _____.

10. Visual examination of the bladder is called _____.

DEFINING ABBREVIATIONS

Define the following abbreviations:

1. C&S _____

_____

2. IVP _____

_____

11. gynecomastia   _____

_____

12. lipids   _____

_____

13. hyperglycemia   _____

_____

14. polydipsia   _____

_____

15. polyuria   _____

_____

16. polyphagia   _____

_____

17. precocious   _____

_____

18. virilism   _____

_____

19. ketoacidosis   _____

_____

20. acromegaly   _____

_____

21. adenoma   _____

_____

22. amenorrhea   _____

_____

23. diabetic retinopathy   _____

_____

24. goiter   _____

_____

25. ketones   _____

_____

MATCHING

Match the abbreviation with the correct definition.

_____ **1.** NIDDM

_____ **2.** ACTH

_____ **3.** TSH

_____ **4.** STH

_____ **5.** MSH

_____ **6.** FSH

_____ **7.** LH

_____ **8.** ICSH

_____ **9.** IDDM

_____ **10.** GH

_____ **11.** ADH

a. somatropic hormone

b. antidiuretic hormone

c. non-insulin-dependent diabetes mellitus

d. follicle-stimulating hormone

e. growth hormone

f. interstitial cell-stimulating hormone

g. adrenocorticotropin hormone

h. insulin-dependent diabetes mellitus

i. thyroid stimulating hormone

j. lutenizing hormone

k. melanocyte stimulating hormone

DEFINING WORD FORMS

Define the following word forms:

1. dipsia _____

_____

2. acro _____

_____

3. pan _____

_____

4. poly _____

_____

5. anti _____

_____

6. di _____

_____

  7. uri

  _____

  _____

  8. adeno

  _____

  _____

  9. oma

  _____

  _____

 10. dys

  _____

  _____

 11. phagia

  _____

  _____

 12. calc

  _____

  _____

 13. hyper

  _____

  _____

 14. glyc

  _____

  _____

 15. hypo

  _____

  _____

 16. retino

  _____

  _____

 17. pathy

  _____

  _____

 18. phagia

  _____

  _____

 19. emia

  _____

  _____

 20. ectomy

  _____

  _____

MATCHING

Match the disease with the correct definition.

_____ 1. hyperpituitarism

_____ 2. Type 1 diabetes

_____ 3. cretinism

_____ 4. Graves' disease

_____ 5. diabetes insipidus

_____ 6. goiter

_____ 7. Cushing's syndrome

_____ 8. Conn's syndrome

_____ 9. Addison's disease

_____ 10. Type 2 diabetes

a. formerly known as juvenile onset diabetes

b. decrease in the release of vasopressin

c. enlargement of the thyroid gland due to inadequate dietary iodine

d. overproduction of aldosterone

e. formerly known as adult onset diabetes

f. abnormal increase in the activity of the pituitary gland

g. hypothyroidism in infants and children

h. overproduction of cortisol

i. hyperthyroidism caused by an autoimmune disorder

j. hypoadrenalism

CONDITION TABLE

Complete the following table:

Condition and Definition	Signs and Symptoms	Diagnostic Tests	Treatment Plan
Goiter			
Diabetes Mellitus			
Diabetes Insipidus			

CONDITION TABLE (continued)

Condition and Definition	Signs and Symptoms	Diagnostic Tests	Treatment Plan
Giantism			
Addison's Disease			
Hypothyroidism			
Hypogonadism			
Conn's Disease			
Hyperparathyroidism			

COMPLETION

Complete the following statements:

1. _____ _____ promotes the growth and development of all body tissues.

2. Hyperpituitarism occurring before puberty is known as _____.

3. Hypopituitarism results in _____.

4. A decrease in the release of vasopressin results in _____.

5. The hormone _____ regulates metabolism.

6. Hyperthyroidism caused by an autoimmune condition is also known as _____.

7. _____ _____ is a life-threatening exacerbation of all symptoms of hyperthyroidism.

8. An enlargement of the thyroid gland due to inadequate dietary iodine is called _____.

9. Hypothyroidism in children is called _____.

10. Low blood calcium levels result in _____.

11. _____ _____ is due to an overproduction of cortisol.

12. Undersecretion of hormones produced by the adrenal cortex is called _____.

13. The two hormones secreted by the pancreas are _____ and _____.

14. When cells burn fats and proteins for energy, they produce a waste product called _____.

15. The condition of having ketones in the blood, breath, and urine is called _____.

16. Three symptoms of diabetes mellitus include _____, _____, and _____.

17. A condition that comes on rapidly as a result of too much insulin is called

_____ _____.

18. _____ _____ is the result of not administer-

ing enough insulin or taking in too many carbohydrates in the diet.

19. _____ _____ is a result of pregnancy.

20. Decreased production of sex hormones results in _____.

SHORT ANSWER

Answer the following questions:

1. List the symptoms of insulin shock.

_____

_____

_____

2. List the symptoms of diabetic coma.

_____

_____

_____

Nervous System Diseases and Disorders

DEFINING TERMS

Define the following terms:

1. dura mater _____

_____

2. arachnoid _____

_____

3. pia mater _____

_____

4. cephalalgia _____

_____

5. sleep apnea _____

_____

6. amnesia _____

_____

7. hypothermia _____

_____

8. insomnia _____

_____

9. chorea _____

_____

10. hydrophobia _____

_____

11. intractable   _____

_____

12. stenosis   _____

_____

13. convulsion   _____

_____

14. seizure   _____

_____

15. concussion   _____

_____

DEFINING ABBREVIATIONS

Define the following abbreviations:

1. CSF   _____

_____

2. TIA   _____

_____

3. CVA   _____

_____

4. CNS   _____

_____

5. PNS   _____

_____

6. ANS   _____

_____

7. HNP   _____

_____

8. EEG   _____

_____

9. ICP _____

_____

10. ALS _____

_____

DEFINING DIAGNOSTIC TESTS

Define the following diagnostic tests:

1. spinal tap/lumbar puncture _____

_____

2. electroencephalogram _____

_____

3. motor testing _____

_____

4. sensory testing _____

_____

5. mental or cognitive testing _____

_____

6. cerebrospinal fluid analysis _____

_____

7. myelogram _____

_____

8. angiograms _____

_____

DEFINING TERMS

Define the following terms:

1. nuchal rigidity _____

_____

2. transient ischemic attacks _____

_____

3. spinal stenosis _____

_____

4. quadriplegia _____

_____

5. paraplegia _____

_____

6. aura _____

_____

7. petit mal seizures _____

_____

8. grand mal seizures _____

_____

9. status epilepticus _____

_____

10. obstructive apnea _____

_____

11. craniotomy _____

_____

12. paresthesia _____

_____

13. pill-rolling motion _____

_____

14. cauterization _____

_____

15. endarterectomy _____

_____

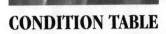

CONDITION TABLE

Complete the following table:

Condition and Definition	Signs and Symptoms	Diagnostic Tests	Treatment Plan
Parkinson's Disease			
Concussion/ Contusion			
Subdural Hematoma			
Meningitis			
Encephalitis			
Shingles			

CONDITION TABLE (continued)

Condition and Definition	Signs and Symptoms	Diagnostic Tests	Treatment Plan
Cerebrovascular Accident			
Transient Ischemic Attacks			
Headaches			
Epilepsy			
Bell's Palsy			
Alzheimer's Disease			
Sleep Apnea			

COMPLETION

Complete the following statements:

1. _____ is another name for headaches.

2. Abnormal muscle contractions are known as _____.

3. _____ means difficult to stop or control.

4. _____ _____ _____ are also called "mini strokes."

5. _____ _____ means without sleep.

6. The inability to fall or stay asleep is called _____.

7. A blow to the head by an object, fall, or other trauma is known as a(n) _____.

8. _____ is loss of memory.

9. An incision into the skull is called _____.

10. _____ is throat spasms caused by the sight of water or attempting to drink water.

11. Constant jerky uncontrollable movement is called _____.

12. _____ is an abnormal sensation, burning, tingling, or numbness.

13. Paralysis of all four extremities is called _____.

14. Inflammation of the brain is called _____.

15. _____ _____ is the inner layer of the meninges.

16. _____ _____ is when the neck resists bending forward or sideways.

17. Paralysis below the waist is called _____.

18. Pill-rolling of the fingers is a classic symptom of _____ _____.

19. The brain and the spinal cord make up the _____ nervous system.

DEFINING DISEASE CONDITIONS

Define the following disease conditions:

1. retinoblastoma _____

   _____

2. Ménière's disease _____

   _____

3. macular degeneration _____

   _____

4. corneal abrasion _____

   _____

5. otitis externa _____

   _____

6. sensorineural deafness _____

   _____

7. motion sickness _____

   _____

8. retinal detachment _____

   _____

DEFINING DIAGNOSTIC TESTS

Define the following diagnostic tests:

1. tonometry _____

   _____

2. angiography _____

   _____

3. audiometry _____

   _____

4. visual acuity _____

   _____

CONDITION TABLE

Complete the following table:

Condition and Definition	Signs and Symptoms	Diagnostic Tests	Treatment Plan
Retinal Detachment			
Otosclerosis			
Diabetic Retinopathy			
Mastoiditis			
Otitis Media			
Ménière's Disease			
Cataracts			

18. prophylactic   _____

_____

19. multiparity   _____

_____

20. primigravid   _____

_____

21. hyperemesis   _____

_____

22. antiemetic   _____

_____

23. proteinuria   _____

_____

24. uterine prolapse   _____

_____

25. ectopic   _____

_____

CONDITION TABLE

Complete the following table:

Disease Condition and Definition	Signs and Symptoms	Diagnostic Tests	Treatment Plan
Transurethral Resection of the Prostate			
Ectopic Pregnancy			

(continued)

CONDITION TABLE (continued)

Disease Condition and Definition	Signs and Symptoms	Diagnostic Tests	Treatment Plan
Hyperemesis Gravidarum			
Abruptio Placentae			
Placenta Previa			
Toxic Shock Syndrome			
Menopause			
Mastectomy			

CONDITION TABLE (continued)

Disease Condition and Definition	Signs and Symptoms	Diagnostic Tests	Treatment Plan
Premenstrual Syndrome			
Endometriosis			

COMPLETION

Complete the following statements:

1. _____ is without menses.

2. Abnormal growth of the lining of the uterus outside the uterus is called

   _____.

3. _____ is painful sexual intercourse.

4. Abnormal bleeding between menstrual periods is called _____.

5. Bad, painful, or difficult menses is known as _____.

6. _____ is excessive or prolonged menstrual bleeding.

7. An X-ray of the uterus and the fallopian tubes is called a _____.

8. A procedure done to look inside the abdominal cavity is called a _____.

9. The study of cells is called _____.

10. The foreskin is known medically as the _____.

11. _____ _____ is commonly known as

    a miscarriage.

12. _____ is excessive vomiting.

13. Another name for toxemia is _____.

14. The medical term for first pregnancy is _____.

15. A pregnancy that occurs when the fertilized ovum attaches outside the uterus is called
_____.

16. Surgical excision of the testes is called a(n) _____.

17. _____ is undescended testicles.

18. Inflammation of the storage tank for sperm is called _____.

19. The slang word for gonorrhea is _____.

20. A painless, highly contagious lesion is called _____.

21. In order to feel the prostate, the physician must perform a _____
_____ _____.

22. A VDRL and an RPR are blood tests performed to test for _____.

23. The natural halting of menstruation is called _____.

24. The surgical excision of the breast is called _____.

25. Inflammation of the cervix is called _____.

Integumentary System Diseases and Disorders

18

COMPLETION

Using the words in the list, complete the following statements:

abrasion	alopecia	avulsion	comedones
contusion	erythema	incision	vesicles
wheals	blunt trauma	laceration	lesion
paronychia	pruritus	pustule	sebum
ulcer	exacerbation		

1. _____ is produced by the sebaceous glands.

2. _____ is the medical term for redness.

3. Severe itching is also known as _____.

4. A broad term meaning abnormality of tissue or any discontinuity is called a(n) _____.

5. A(n) _____ is a small circumscribed elevation of the skin containing pus.

6. A small solid raised lesion less than 0.5 cm in diameter is called a _____.

7. A _____ is an open sore or erosion of the skin or mucous membrane.

8. A smooth, slightly elevated swollen area that is redder or paler than the surrounding skin is usually accompanied by itching is known as a(n) _____.

9. A(n) _____ is a plugged skin pore.

10. A type of sebaceous cyst is called a _____ _____.

11. Bacterial infection of the nails is called a(n) _____.

12. A common mechanical injury caused by scraping away the skin surface is called a(n)
_____.

13. A(n) _____ occurs when a portion of skin or an appendage is
pulled or torn away.

14. A cut in the skin caused by a sharp object such as a knife, razor, or glass is known
medically as a(n) _____.

15. When an individual is struck by items such as hammers or clubs or is thrown into objects
like a steering wheel and walls, the individual may sustain a _____
_____ injury.

DEFINING TERMS

Define the following terms:

1. epidermis _____
_____

2. sebum _____
_____

3. keratin _____
_____

4. lesions _____
_____

5. pruritus _____
_____

6. erythema _____
_____

7. vesicles _____
_____

8. pustules _____
_____

11. phenotype _____

12. recessive _____

13. stricture _____

14. viscous _____

15. polydactyly _____

16. dystrophy _____

17. hydrocephalus _____

18. chordee _____

19. epispadias _____

20. anomaly _____

DEFINING ABBREVIATIONS

Define the following abbreviations:

1. FAS _____

2. PKU _____

3. CP _____

4. CHD _____

_____

5. MD _____

_____

DEFINING DIAGNOSTIC TESTS

Define the following diagnostic tests:

1. amniotic fluid analysis _____

_____

2. ultrasonography _____

_____

3. muscle biopsy _____

_____

4. electromyography _____

_____

5. blood test for phenylketonuria _____

_____

CONDITION TABLE

Complete the following table:

Condition and Definition	Signs and Symptoms	Diagnostic Tests	Treatment Plan
Tay-Sachs Disease			
Fetal Alcohol Syndrome			

CONDITION TABLE (continued)

Condition and Definition	Signs and Symptoms	Diagnostic Tests	Treatment Plan
Hirschsprung's Disease			
Down Syndrome			
Phenylketonuria			
Failure to Thrive			
Imperforate Anus			
Cleft Palate			

(continued)

CONDITION TABLE (continued)

Condition and Definition	Signs and Symptoms	Diagnostic Tests	Treatment Plan
Tetralogy of Fallot			
Meckel's Diverticulum			

COMPLETION

Complete the following statements:

1. Babies born with tetralogy of Fallot are called _____

    _____.

2. An abnormality is known as a(n) _____.

3. A condition a person is born with is known as _____.

4. An abnormal heart sound is called a(n) _____.

5. _____ is a small brain.

6. The process of visualizing chromosomes is called _____.

7. _____ is listening to the chest with a stethoscope.

8. Being in control means being in _____.

9. _____ are also called sex cells.

10. The expression of a trait such as brown hair or blue eyes is called a(n)

    _____.

CONDITION TABLE (continued)

Condition and Definition	Signs and Symptoms	Diagnostic Tests	Treatment Plan
Measles			
Mumps			
Rubella			
Pertussis			
Diphtheria			
AIDS			
Croup			
Tuberculosis			

COMPLETION

Complete the following statements:

1. Another name for measles is _____.

2. Pertussis is also called _____.

3. An infection of the parotid glands is known as _____.

4. An inflammation of the testes is called _____.

5. _____ is more commonly called flu.

6. _____ are unique to measles and are often the definitive symptoms that make the diagnosis.

7. _____ is excessive gas.

8. _____ are blister-like eruptions on the skin.

9. Inflammation of the nasal mucous membranes is called _____.

10. _____ is a feeling of general discomfort.

11. The _____ _____ is the time between exposure to the disease and the presence of the symptoms that lasts several days.

12. _____ _____ is a high-pitched sound during inspiration due to a blocked airway.

13. _____ is a spasm or convulsion.

14. _____ is the state of being inactive.

15. _____ are lice eggs.

16. _____ is lying face down.

17. _____ is lying face up.

18. Rabbit fever is also known as _____.

19. _____ is also known as croup.

20. A crossed or lazy eye is called _____.

Mental Health Diseases and Disorders

DEFINING TERMS

Define the following terms:

1. addiction _____

_____

2. affect _____

_____

3. bulimia _____

_____

4. delirium tremens _____

_____

5. circadian rhythms _____

_____

6. delusions _____

_____

7. dependency _____

_____

8. intoxicated _____

_____

9. mania _____

_____

10. mood _____

_____

11. obsession _____

_____

12. organic _____

_____

13. tolerance _____

_____

14. stuttering _____

_____

15. enuresis _____

_____

16. tics _____

_____

17. narcotics _____

_____

18. psychosis _____

_____

19. schizophrenia _____

_____

20. grandiose _____

_____

21. jealous _____

_____

22. persecutory _____

_____

23. somatic _____

_____

24. depersonalization _____

_____

25. conversion _____

_____

26. malingering _____

_____